Green Smoothie Bible: The Complete Smoothie Cleanse Guide

Are Green Smoothies Really Good For You?

By: Patricia Young

Publishers Notes

Disclaimer

This publication is intended to provide helpful and informative material. It is not intended to diagnose, treat, cure, or prevent any health problem or condition, nor is intended to replace the advice of a physician. No action should be taken solely on the contents of this book. Always consult your physician or qualified health-care professional on any matters regarding your health and before adopting any suggestions in this book or drawing inferences from it.

The author and publisher specifically disclaim all responsibility for any liability, loss or risk, personal or otherwise, which is incurred as a consequence, directly or indirectly, from the use or application of any contents of this book.

Any and all product names referenced within this book are the trademarks of their respective owners. None of these owners have sponsored, authorized, endorsed, or approved this book.

Always read all information provided by the manufacturers' product labels before using their products. The author and publisher are not responsible for claims made by manufacturers.

Digital Edition

Manufactured in the United States of America

WHAT YOU WILL LEARN IN THIS BOOK

How This Book Will Help You and Why

If you have ever wondered if a green smoothie is really good for you then you need to keep on reading this book. It will not only explain what a smoothie is and how to make a basic smoothie but it goes into in-depth explanations of the various ways that a smoothie can benefit the body.

In addition to that there are a few teaser recipes that users can try to see how tasty these green smoothie recipes can be.

Dive Right into the Book! Or Learn a Bit More About the Author

TABLE OF CONTENTS

CHAPTER 1- SMOOTHIES- AN OVERVIEW

Everyone has those days. You feel limp and lifeless and do not burn ahead. You have no energy and there seems to be no end to the ay. Unfortunately, we assume wrongly that this kind of day is simply unavoidable, while the solution is amazingly simple. Making a green smoothie! From this countless people feel they are healthier, more vital and prepared to go through life. Every day!

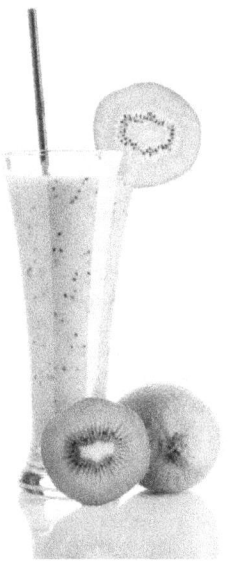

Making a smoothie with fruit? Having a limp and lifeless feeling is caused by a deficiency of vitamins and minerals. By drinking a green smoothie daily you absorb nutrients easier and right away you'll have more energy. All you need is a blender, leafy vegetables (spinach, lettuce or endive), fruit, water and a few minutes of your time. The fruit makes the smoothie a nice sweet drink that may be drunk by everyone and is ideal for those who do not like to eat vegetables!

Daily green smoothie making will ensure that you have enough energy every day. A green smoothie also makes for a better immune system and has a positive effect on blood pressure and bowel movements. You super fit all day and your skin will shine again.

In addition, a green smoothie is ideal for weight maintenance or weight loss. Green smoothies give a sense of satisfaction through which overeating is prevented. Daily green smoothie making provides your body with the necessary vitamins and minerals.

Green smoothies are harmless! The only adverse effect a green smoothie can have in the beginning is that the body will detoxify. You will get so many nutrients that the body will get rid of existing toxins. This is precisely what makes you healthier and more radiant will go through life.

CHAPTER 2- ADDING WHEATGRASS TO YOUR SMOOTHIE

As popular as weight loss smoothies have become recently, this is a question that you will probably encounter at some point in your smoothie-making career if you are serious about making smoothies. So why don't we take a look at whether or not adding wheatgrass to your smoothies is a good idea. But first, what exactly is wheat grass?

Wheatgrass is on it's own a complete food that can be grown from the sprout of a wheat berry, which as it turns out is the seed or kernel of the common wheat plant. It belongs to the cereal grass family. You might recognize it's other family members as rye grass, oat grass and barley. Usually it's harvested when the wheatgrass is at its highest peak in nutritional value and is loaded with vitamins, nutrients, amino acids, antioxidants etc. The reason why it's harvested at this point is because once the wheatgrass fully matures you won't be able to find all of those nutrients in it. What you need to look out for is that it is a dark green color and looks similar to the grass you would find in your lawn.

While we are on the subject of wheatgrass, let's talk about some of the benefits that can come from adding it to your smoothies. With wheatgrass as a part of your smoothie regimen, you could start to see things like:

- Stronger and healthier nails and hair

- Fewer skin problems
- Improved energy levels
- Weight loss
- Improved mental clarity
- Feeling fuller longer
- Fewer problems with acid reflux

How Can I Add Wheatgrass To My Smoothie?

Okay, so you are sold on using the wheatgrass, but how do you add it to your smoothie. You might be tempted to simply throw it in your blender with the other ingredients. If you did that, you would be wrong. I would highly recommend that when you decide to add it to your shake, you do so in the juice form and not in its whole form. The reason being once you put it into your blender it becomes much harder for you to be able to extract all of the nutrients that it has. You may be able to get some of the nutrients using a more powerful high speed blender, but that's a lot of work for so little nutrients.

Getting Wheatgrass In The Juice Form

The easiest way for you to get the vital juices from your wheatgrass is by using a juicer. I know, it sounds really hard. Once you have the juice you can then add that to your smoothie.

Alternatives To Using Wheatgrass

As with any smoothie that you make, there are different alternatives that you can use if you don't like using wheatgrass. That would include spinach, kale, broccoli etc. I would suggest that you mix things up a bit so that you won't get used to or bored with using the same ingredient over and over.

What If You Are Allergic To Wheatgrass?

If this is the case, then there is a big chance that what you are allergic to is gluten. You can read more about gluten-free smoothies to learn more about them. But in a nutshell, gluten is formed in the actual wheat grain and wheatgrass is harvested and cut before it develops a seed head. So this would make the wheatgrass juice gluten-free.

There you have it. You have just learned that you can indeed have a healthy smoothie loaded with wheatgrass.

CHAPTER 3- WHY DO SMOOTHIES TURN BROWN

If you are like me, then you have made your fair share of smoothies. I've used God knows how many different ingredients over the years along with a number of different combinations. In doing so, I've come across some different color combinations that would make you take a second look and also question what was going on.

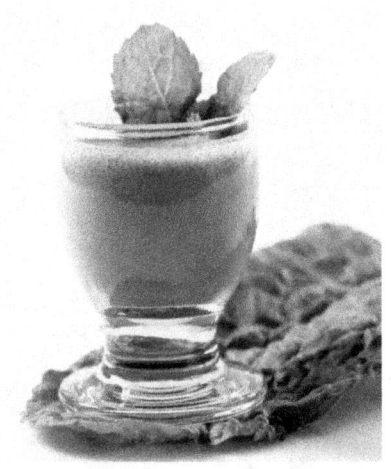

However, before you get all worked up over it; let's determine exactly why you may see your smoothie turn brown on you. But first, does the color have any effect on the nutrient value of your smoothie? Absolutely not. The color of your smoothie is basically there for cosmetic reasons. You will still get all of the vitamins and nutrients that all of the fruits and veggies have. Some people are turned off by certain colors when it comes to their foods and drinks. If this is you, then I will show you how to get past this issue.

Now let's take a look at what causes your smoothies to turn brown. Typically you will find that your smoothies will turn green when you are making, wait for it...the green smoothies. Here's how it happens.

Remember way back when you were a kid in grade school and your really smart teacher was going over the colors in the color chart. He/she would say things like yellow + blue = green. Do you remember that? The reason why your smoothie is turning brown has to do with the colors that you are mixing together. If you mix red plus green you will get the color brown. And therein lays your issue.

But where does the color red come from? It comes from the use of red strawberries mixed with green veggies. When you use fruits that are more of the color white like a banana, you won't get the brown final color. It's only when you combine the green with the red do you get a tasty brown drink.

Changing The Color

By now I think you get the idea of how the color brown comes about in your smoothies as well as the simple remedy to fix it.

All that you have to do is to use a different fruit combination with the veggies. If you don't like the thought of downing a brown smoothie, then you could substitute fruits that are lighter in color.

CHAPTER 4- DO SMOOTHIES GIVE YOU GAS?

One of the questions I get asked a lot is "Why do smoothies give me gas?" Actually, this is a very common problem. You'll see it quite often when you are making a sudden change to your diet (especially if you are switching to using green smoothies). The important thing to note here is that bloating can be caused by a variety of different things. It can be caused by certain foods or from having a medical condition.

I just want to stress here that because of the many possibilities that can cause you to suffer from gas, there is no way I can cover each and every one of them here in this chapter. So what I will do instead is cover some of the most common reasons why you might suffer from bloating immediately after drinking your smoothie.

Okay, so let's say that you don't have any medical issues going on with your body, and by that I mean that your doctor has not said that you have any particular ailments that you currently suffer from. No indigestion or anything like that. From there let's assume that you experience the bloating only after you have drank a green smoothie or you've taken in quite a bit more fruit than you would normally eat. If this doesn't sound like you then please make sure you check in with your doctor as I am not using this chapter as a way to give you medical advice. Over the years, when I've seen this type of situation happen, it is usually has two causes.

Too Much, Too Soon

You might love to eat fruit, and you might love to drink your green smoothies, but the problem here is that there is such a situation as too much of a good thing (its also one of the unfortunate drawbacks to drinking green smoothies). If you find that your recipe calls for making an eight ounce shake, and you're putting in twenty ounces, then guess what. You're getting too much too soon. This is especially true if your body is not used to getting so much fiber so fast. The sudden introduction of a lot of fruit and fiber into your diet can put your body into a form of shock. If you overload your body's ability to breakdown and digest fructose (it's the sugar that can be found in fruit) then some of that fructose can actually remain in your digestive tract. From there it can begin to ferment and start to produce gas. You'll know this by the uncomfortable feeling that will accompany this process.

How do you fix it? Well, not to sound sarcastic here, your solution is simple. Cut back on how much you drink. I know, real earth shattering right. But it goes without saying that if you make a 32 ounce pitcher and in so doing, it gives you terrible stomach problems; then you should try drinking 8 ounces. From there you would work your way back up to guzzling the 32 ounces over time.

You have to find your tolerance level. It may be 8 ounces, it may be 16 ounces. You have to experiment with it to know for sure. Also, keep in mind that if you continue to have problems even after making these changes, then you might want to consult your doctor to get checked out for a condition called fructose malabsorption.

Getting Too Much Fat Mixed In With Your Fruit

This is the second cause that can lead you to feeling like you are bloated after you've drank a green smoothie. The reason for this is that you have too much fat being mixed in with fruit. Your body will digest fruits at a much faster rate than it digests fats from sources like nuts or seeds. Giving your body too much fat too fast can lead to you having a lot of gas.

Think of it like this. If you eat a meal that is high in fat and then follow that up with some fruit, then what will happen is the fat you've just eaten will digest slowly and in the meantime the fruit will get held up in your intestines and start to ferment. Because of this you will feel and look like a balloon that's about to explode.

CHAPTER 5- ARE SMOOTHIES HEALTHY FOR DIABETICS?

If you were to ask 10 people "Are smoothies healthy for diabetics?"...You would probably get 10 different answers. And the reason for that is because there is a lot of information out there for people to choose from and not all of it is true. So I am going to try to clear up some of the confusion.

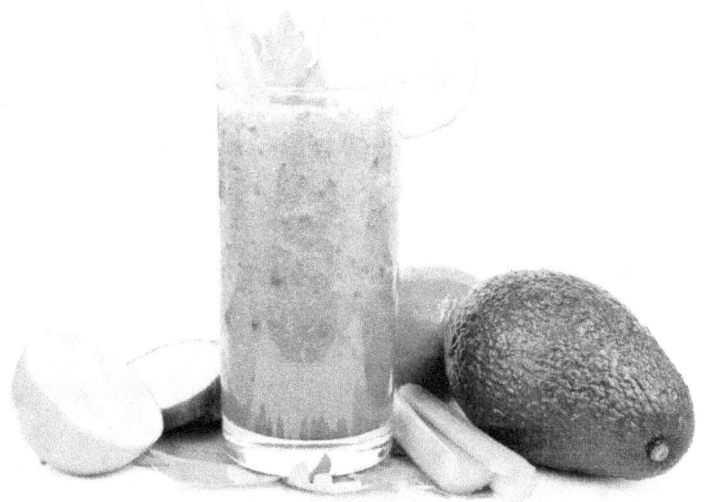

First up, why are smoothies considered to be bad for diabetics? Part of this reasoning comes from the belief that the sugars that are contained in the fruits themselves are sweet. However, most fruits are okay for a diabetic diet. You could consider apples, berries, kiwi and mangos. These fruits in particular don't contain fructose, so they don't mess with your body's dependence on insulin.

If you are diabetic, then you can consider using apples in a smoothie, because apples contain pectin which helps in lowering your blood glucose levels.

Fruits That You Shouldn't Use In Your Smoothies If You Are A Diabetic

I should also mention that just as apples are a good fruit to use in your smoothies if you are diabetic, there are some other fruits that you should avoid. Those fruits would be grapes, watermelons, and oranges as these fruits can elevate your blood sugar levels.

But what happens if you want to use a dairy product like milk? It is not a done deal for you if you want to use milk in your smoothies. What you can do instead is use soy milk. When you use soy milk you are adding protein and calcium to your drink and will give your drink a creamy consistency; unlike its counterpart, whole milk, which can add saturated fats which can do a number on your bad cholesterol levels and increase your risk of diabetes related heart disease. Also, if you happen to be allergic to soy you can choose skim milk or opt for fat free milk instead.

Okay, so what's an alternative to using fruits if you are diabetic? The answer here for you would be to use veggies. It's true that most smoothies consist of fruits. However, you can use veggies to boost up the nutrition content of your smoothies. You will want to use vegetables that are high in fiber which in turn can help you with managing your blood glucose levels.

If you are diabetic, you can still make yourself a smoothie as long as you pay attention to the types of fruits that you use and opt for more veggies in your drink.

CHAPTER 6- ARE SMOOTHIES SAFE DURING PREGNANCY?

Many women who are pregnant and who want to keep their weight down during their pregnancy often wonder if it's okay to use smoothies during their pregnancy. As it turns out, there are some things you should know if you are currently thinking about adding smoothies to your diet plans.

One of the big questions that women have about using smoothies during their pregnancy is whether or not the smoothies will affect their baby or the health of their baby. There isn't any current study that discusses the effect that drinking smoothies during your pregnancy would have on your baby.

However, there is quite a bit of evidence that shows that drinking smoothies during your pregnancy can have an effect on you the mother. In particular they can make you sick. We all know that mothers can get morning sickness which usually comes during the first trimester of their pregnancy. The major issue being the nausea associated with that trimester. One way for expecting mothers to deal with this is by making sure that they keep food in their stomachs. Smoothies of course offer an easier way to do that, rather than struggling with trying to get normal cooked food down your throat. They also offer an easy way to get nutrients into your system. Just keep in mind that if you do choose to drink a smoothie, make sure that you stay away from aromatic fruits as well as full fat dairy products because the scent of these items can make your morning sickness even worse and you really don't want to do that.

Smoothies That Can Harm You During Your Pregnancy

There is a certain type of smoothie that can really have a dramatic effect on your pregnancy if you are not careful. This smoothie is the one that is made with unpasteurized juices which is truly dangerous to expecting moms. I know that you might be thinking where in the heck you would get unpasteurized juices. Well you normally can get them from local farmers markets or fruit stands. The juices sold there, although tasty, they have not been through the process of high temperature heating to kill any dangerous microbes that might be in the juices. You have to make sure that you take care and wash off any fruits that you get from either farmers markets or fruit stands and put off using any unpasteurized juices.

What About Purchasing Fruit Smoothies?

Well if you're thinking about purchasing a smoothie from a store, than I would recommend that you hold off on that. The reason being, you don't always know what's inside of that smoothie that you are getting from the store. When you make your own smoothies you know exactly what's going into them and can control the calories and sugars much better. I would also recommend that you use strawberries in your smoothie if you choose to use them during your pregnancy, because the strawberry has lower sugar than many other fruits.

Chapter 7- Smoothies- Are They A Good Choice For Losing Weight?

Is there any truth to the saying that weight loss smoothies can be used for losing weight as well as giving you better health and even helping you with certain skin conditions that you might have? That's the question I'll answer for you in this chapter. However, first, imagine this for a moment. You want to lose some weight and you are up in arms about the additional pounds that can now be seen around your waistline and the silly remarks and laughter that come from your friends and family. You've probably also heard about how you can use weight loss smoothies to burn off stubborn fat without having to go on some crazy crash diet. But one question still remains. Are diet shakes and weight loss smoothies your best option when it comes to weight loss?

Maybe you are wondering if you can actually use weight loss smoothies to lose weight fast without any kind of pills and if these beverages can actually help you attain a flat belly. In fact, many people are left in awe as to how these sweet-tasting beverages actually help you if you are struggling with losing weight to achieve a slimmer body shape. There is no hiding the fact that pre-packaged smoothie weight loss drinks are arguably the best option specifically designed to assist you in dropping those extra pounds due to their low calorie intake. However, are there any real benefits?

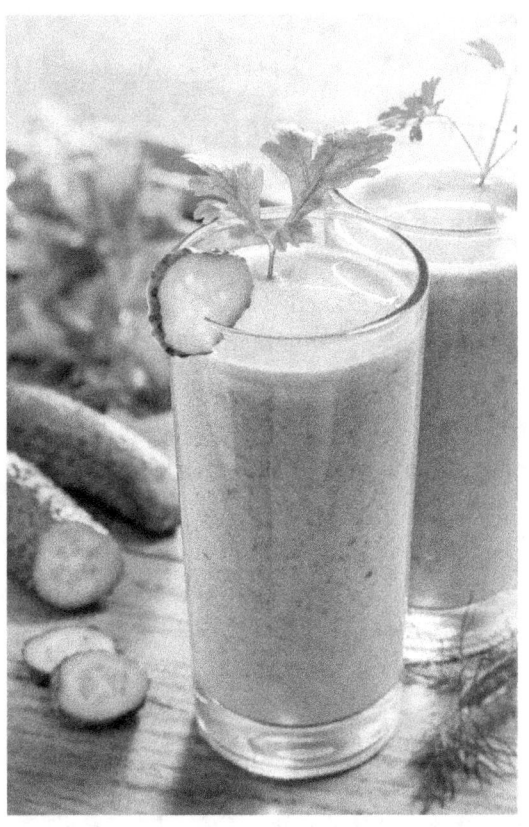

The answer is yes! Weight loss smoothies do come with their fair share of benefits. The fact that these beverages are full of nutritional value means their intake gives your body much needed nutrition on a regular basis. As a result, they remain a go to source in helping you achieve your goal of trimming down your body weight much more easily. In my opinion, the reason why they are so valuable is that more often than not, they are created using fresh fruits or vegetables and because of that, they help ensure that your body receives the vital nutrition it requires.

It is very difficult to find any of the over-counter snacks that contain both vitamins and minerals. For every rule that you have though, there is always an exception and a smoothie is the real exception in this case. Believe it or not, it is one of the few over-the-counter snacks that are easy to make yourself and effective to use. They are the perfect solution if your main goal is to burn off unwanted fat.

Another benefit you get from weight loss smoothies is that more often than not, the smoothies are pre-portioned. For you, the work is already cut out in terms of not having to dedicate so much of your time towards getting them ready for intake. Many people hardly appreciate this feature. Indeed, the fact that they are portioned-out already helps you to regulate your daily calorie intake. A pre-portioned product helps you follow your daily diet plan. You will not consume above the required levels.

Something else for you to consider about the beauty of low calorie weight loss smoothies is that they are portioned out to satisfy your attempts towards losing weight on a regular basis. When you adopt a diet plan to burn fat, preparing a smoothie on your own at home may result in a drink full of too many calories. The issue then becomes, if you consume a lot of it, how much will you be interfering with your diet plans. Therefore, the right quantity is vital to promote the shedding of those unwanted pounds.

There are several low calorie weight loss smoothies mostly containing vegetables or fruits to choose from. Vegetable smoothies contain low calories and offer your body quite a few health benefits. Additionally, they can also help to prevent several body diseases such as liver disease, high cholesterol as well as diabetes. In fact when you use a green smoothie regimen, it's fair to say that you can see a dramatic drop in your overall cholesterol numbers.

And yet there's something else you should know about the benefits of meal replacement smoothies. They taste great! When they say you can't drink just one, they really aren't kidding. I love making my weight loss smoothies in such a way that they curb my appetite. And although I love them when I use fruit, I generally tend to experience more calories being burned when I use the vegetable smoothies. You might find the same to be true for you as well. You'll have to do a little experimenting to find out.

If you still doubt whether or not you should use weight loss smoothies on a regular basis, then the information that you will find here should be of help to you. Smoothies are one of the best options in respect to burning extra body fat. As a result, they are often referred to as meal replacements and are often substituted when you have to skip meals. Given that the majority of people have tight schedules nowadays; they serve as the perfect meal replacements. If your mornings are crazy and you always miss breakfast, a gulp on your way to work is recommended. Given that they can curb your appetite, hunger shouldn't be an issue. The taste and texture offered by these drinks might take some getting used to, however don't overlook the nutritional value that makes them vital for your well-being. This is definitely the right product for those looking to enjoy the process of trimming down body weight.

CHAPTER 8- HOW TO MAKE A HEALTHY FRUIT SMOOTHIE FOR BREAKFAST

If you are like me, then that means you actually like having a healthy fruit smoothie for breakfast. It serves as a way to get your day off to a good start. But before you can even do that you first have to know how to make a great tasting smoothie. And so we are going to go over how you can do just that.

What Actually Makes A Healthy Fruit Smoothie?

As it turns out what really makes them healthy comes down to a number of things. One being that you are using fruits in their natural form and because of that, although your smoothie will still have some calories that come from sugar, it will come in its most natural form and not the processed version. Plus by using the fruits in your smoothie it will also give you your daily recommended requirements.

You can also add other ingredients that are both healthy and come loaded with different vitamins and nutrients. Things like yogurt, almond milk, flax seeds etc.

Another benefit of having a healthy fruit smoothie for breakfast is that it can help reduce your risk of heart disease. The more servings you have, the lower your risks become.

Can A Healthy Fruit Smoothie Be Used As A Meal Replacement?

This is a common question that's asked, and the answer is yes! Of course you can use them as meal replacements. Fruit smoothies can replace either breakfast, lunch or dinner. So don't get caught up in whether or not you should only have your smoothies for lunch or dinner.

Just keep in mind that if you do choose to use your smoothie as a meal replacement, you will have to add a few more ingredients to it than what you might normally have. Primarily you will want to focus on adding protein to your smoothie if you are using it as a meal replacement. You will also want to make sure that you also get some form of fat added to your drink as well because your body will need to have a source of energy. Since you would be replacing a meal, on a daily basis you would normally get between 750 -800 calories for one meal. Obviously you don't want your shake to have those many calories, but you still need the fat so that your body can function as it should.

Now once you decide that you are going to have a healthy fruit smoothie for breakfast as a meal replacement, your choice of protein will become an important factor. I usually recommend that you use pure protein powders if you are using this as your protein source. And by pure protein I mean that the powder shouldn't have too many additional chemicals added to it in order to add more nutrients to it.

How Difficult Is It To Make A Healthy Fruit Smoothie?

It really goes without saying that making your fruit smoothies isn't hard at all. I'll give you the easy way to make them and a way that will require a bit more time on your part, but is still very doable.

The easiest way to make your shakes is to first start off with the right equipment. I can't stress to you enough, how important this is if you are going to make smoothies a regular part of your life. When I first started using smoothies, I didn't have the right blender. It took me much longer to make my shakes and it led to me becoming frustrated at times because I wanted the smoothie but I didn't want to spend all of the time on prepping. When I bit the bullet and purchased a Braun Powermax blender, all of my issues went away. You'll make your smoothies so much faster with a machine like that. However, that speed and ease of use comes with a price though. I had to shell out over $430 for my blender. It's a lot of cash when you see other blenders that promise to do the same thing. But after trying the Oster blender, the Ninja and a couple of others, I didn't get the results that I was looking for from those machines.

What makes having the right equipment the easy way to make your smoothies is that you won't have to spend so much time on preparation. You can put the whole banana in, with the strawberries and blueberries. Before I would have to spend time chopping up the ingredients because the motor couldn't handle processing the larger pieces all at once.

Now for the way that's a bit more time consuming but still doable is to use a lower horsepower blender. Again, here you will have to do a little prep work ahead of time in order to make it easier on your blender. By cutting your fruit up into smaller pieces you will be able to save your motor from burning out too fast because it's working so hard to blend your ingredients.

Alternatives To A Healthy Breakfast Smoothie

If you find that you are in need of an alternative to having a fruit smoothie then I would recommend that you try a meal replacement bar. Keep in mind though that with these bars you have to be mindful of the calories as they can be loaded with sugars.

Below are two breakfast smoothie recipes

Honeydew Kiwi Fruit Smoothie

- 2 cups of honeydew
- 1 kiwi fruit cut up and peeled
- 2 tablespoons of sugar
- 1 small granny smith apple peeled and diced without the core
- 1 cup of ice cubes
- 1 tablespoon of lemon juice

Put the ingredients into a blender and blend together

Banana And Kiwi Smoothie

- 1 kiwi peeled and sliced
- 1 banana, peeled and diced into small chunks

- ½ cup of ice cubes
- 1 cup of low fat yogurt
- 2 table spoons of maple syrup optional

CHAPTER 9- RAW FOOD SMOOTHIES

Nobody is the same. What works for me might not work exactly the same for you. For example, I might add flax seeds to my green smoothie and have no ill effects. No bloating, no gas, nothing. But you on the other hand, after drinking such a combination might blow up. If that's the case, then your solution is to switch over to a simple smoothie. Try it out for a week. You very well may be allergic to certain fruit combinations. Or even to acidic citrus. The point here is that you want to find out for sure.

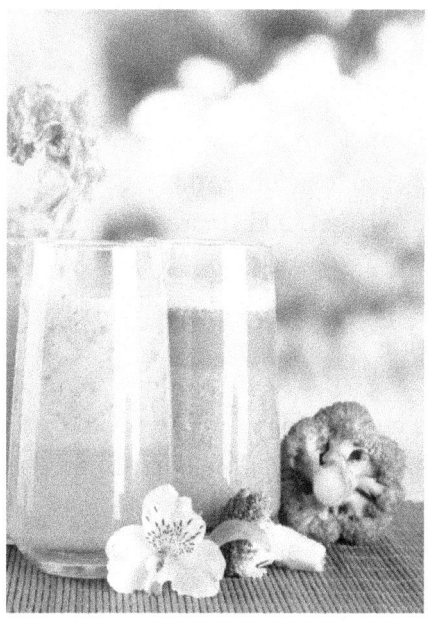

A helpful tip for you is to make sure that you drink your green smoothie by itself and to make sure you don't eat anything for at least two hours before, and two hours after. A good rule of thumb is to have your shake first thing in the morning or as a snack. As much as I'd like to say that every fruit will work for everybody, that's just not the case. You will have to find out what works for your body as I can't tell you what will or won't work for you.

When it comes to changing your diet, there will no doubt be some digestive issues. This is actually normal so don't get scared. Most of the time it will go away on its own as your body gets used to what you are now doing.

You can keep a food journal to keep track of what is working and for what isn't working. That is where you will learn of any intolerance's you might have. If you continue to have digestive issue then you will need to consult your doctor.

A "raw food smoothie" is some fruit and a whole lot of other raw ingredients. The fruit helps mask the taste of other raw ingredients that wouldn't taste very good blended by themselves. This is different from a "green smoothie", because it adds more than just fruit and leafy greens. You will most likely use raw foods that you intuitively like, but it's also a way to consume a variety of raw foods that you don't like much - but you know are really healthy.

Note: I rarely make two raw food smoothies exactly the same. I'm always experimenting with new ingredients. The recipe for a raw food smoothie is only limited by your imagination. In five years, I've only made one I couldn't finish. As long as you include enough fruit, the fruit will mask that taste of anything you don't like.

A typical raw food smoothie recipe:

- About fourteen to sixteen ounces of liquid base. This could be water/coconut water/raw homemade almond milk, etc. Vary the amount of liquid for your personal preference for thickness.

- Banana, or any fruit of your choice: I regularly use mangos, strawberries, peaches, apples, oranges, tangerines, grapefruit, grapes, kiwi, goji berries, etc
- About ½ orange or apple. I usually use two fruits, because I always have several fruits available. Again, any 2nd fruit of your choice.
- ½ avocado. I usually make two drinks at a time, so ½ avocado in each drink.
- Baby carrots 2-4
- Tomatoes: about 3-5 cherry size, or half a golf ball size
- Couple tablespoons of pumpkin seeds (I pre-make mine in the evening for the next day, so the seeds start the sprouting process, which helps unlock it's nutrition).
- Couple tablespoon sunflower kernels (again, soaked overnight).
- Bell pepper (red/orange/yellow) cut small section out, about a cracker in size,
- Shot glass amount of cold pressed virgin olive oil (or oil of your choice).
- Pecans - about 8-10 (substitute walnuts, almonds, etc.).
- Celery - one to two stalks.
- Cucumber - about an inch section.
- Nori (sea vegetable) - about a cracker size of the non-toasted sheet (good for salt and minerals).
- Handful of green leafy vegetable of your choice (spinach, kale, collard greens, romaine lettuce, red chard, etc.). Fresh grown sprouts can also be used. You can use other greens with a really strong taste, but be prepared for unusual flavors that will result. For example, Arugula will add an interesting twang to the drink. Also, be careful about putting too much green leafy stuff in your drink the first time. If the drink is too green, it will taste too green and start to give you that nauseous feeling when you start to drink it (at least for beginners). If that happens, back off by half

the amount of greens and start adding more each day until you get the most greens in your drink without it tasting bad. Eventually, you will intuitively be able to determine how much leafy green to add. Your tolerance for a more green drink will grow over time.

Other optional ingredients I've used: chia seeds, ground flax seed, hemp protein powder, wheat germ powder, raw oat flakes, daikon, radishes, spirulina, bee pollen, and fresh squeezed lime or lemon to add some sweetness.

CHAPTER 10- 3 TASTY SMOOTHIE RECIPES

Fruit Smoothies With Yogurt

A yogurt is basically custard-like food made from curdled milk. There are many types of recipes that can be created using yogurt. A Fruit smoothie with yogurt is one of the most popular drinks that can be prepared using the yogurt. Creating a fruit smoothie with yogurt is not only just easy to prepare, but it is a widely popular drink in many parts of the world. The reason for the immense popularity of this drink is due to the fact that it has a very unique taste and flavor. These types of drinks can be found in all the popular coffee shops and restaurants and even can be made at home.

A smoothie is basically a drink which has a higher density than that of other cold drinks and it is generally made from fruits. It is a blended and very sweet beverage which creates a very refreshing feeling after the drink. Not only just fruit a smoothie can be prepared by using only fruits but it can also be prepared by using chocolates, peanut butter, honey, sweet syrup, milk, ice cream ingredients and even yogurt. This type of drink is very popular among health conscious people from all across the globe. This type has gained immense popularity especially with the United States of America during the 1990's. By the start of the year 2000 this drink became so popular that it could be found in almost the restaurants and popular cafe shops. Among the fruit smoothie the pineapple smoothie and the banana smoothie were very much popular especially in the western countries like United States of America and many European countries. Another very popular fruit smoothie was the smoothie which was prepared using yogurt as its ingredient. Preparing this kind of smoothie is very simple and easy and this kind of smoothies can be created by anyone in his/her home.

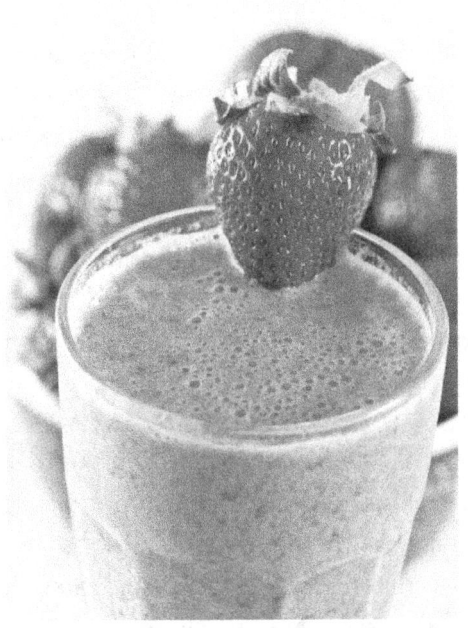

Fruit smoothies with yogurt are a very popular drink in many countries around the world. The main ingredients which are required in order yogurt fruit smoothies are:

- 2 cups of yogurt with vanilla flavor or any other fruit flavor.
- 1 completely cut banana.
- 4 to 5 fresh strawberries are required and it is better if the strawberries are frozen with ice.
- ½ tea spoon of vanilla or almond extract.
- 1 tea spoon of sugar or according to one's desire.

- Lots and lots of ice cubes.

And finally all the main ingredients should be blended gently to prepare the drink.

Raspberry-Colada Smoothie

Fiesta time! There's nothing like a sweet, tropical smoothie. Pina coladas are my favorite, and a touch of sugar-free raspberry syrup (like the ones from Torani) makes this creamy smoothie even better. Here are the ingredients:

- 8 oz. sugar-free lemonade
- 1/2 large, frozen banana, diced
- 1 oz. of frozen pineapple tidbits
- 1/4 t. rum extract

Place all ingredients in blender. Blend. Top with fat-free whipped cream and a bit of fat-free raspberry syrup.

Smoothie Recipes For Kids

Smoothies are snacks for children which are healthy. Smoothie recipes for kids are important owing to the numerous benefits of smoothies; they not only satisfy hunger but also quench thirst. They have a pretty and bright taste; antioxidants and more fibers go to the body as the kid enjoys the taste; fussy ingredients are not needed; smoothies give fruits that are overripe, a another life; smoothie recipes for kids can be customized to suit kid's needs. Green smoothies are made from fresh or leafy greens. These smoothies are appropriate for kids because they feel good and have nutritional supplements in plenty.

One idea of smoothie recipes for kids comprises of bananas, spinach, mangoes, berries, parsley and romaine lettuce. Agave nectar or molasses will make the greener smoothie to be sweeter. A variety of greens can also be used which include Beet Greens, spinach, kale, Collard, romaine and mustard turnip. In such smoothie recipes for kids, include your kid's favorite fruits and using water, mix the drink properly. You can mix greens with anything so no need for fretting about food combination. For children who are into milk, try to mix in some. Tender coconut gives green smoothies a grand taste.

Smoothie recipes for kids may comprise of spinach/baby spinach, chia seeds, peaches, pineapple, frozen bananas, spirulina powder and water. Green smoothies are of great benefit to the kids since they are in liquid form therefore vitamins are minerals are effortlessly taken up into the body. Consequently, when the kid's body has the required nutrients, it will have the right stamina during its daily activities. Not every child is comfortable with these green smoothie recipes for kids, give the mixtures some names or add berries for the flavor to be emphasized.

Utilize natural factors only when introducing these smoothies to your kids. The children will not become fed up if fresh ingredients are included in smoothie recipes for kids. With children, use frozen fruits instead of ice cubes. Before you freeze bananas, they need to be peeled and cut into small pieces. For more nutrients with the green smoothie recipes for kids, milk, yogurt, wheat germs, flax seeds are added to the blender. Some fruits are naturally sweet so sugar will not always be needed. Immediately after using a blender, rinse it because if the fruits and greens dry in it cleaning might be quite difficult.

CHAPTER 11- THE BEST BLENDER FOR MAKING SMOOTHIES

In this our final chapter I will take a look at the best blender for making smoothies at home. Today a good quality kitchen blender is vital to any well equipped kitchen. They are very useful for a wide variety of applications. Whether it is crushing ice or blending soups the blender is one of the most versatile tools in the kitchen. One of the most useful roles a blender can carry out is the blending of homemade smoothies.

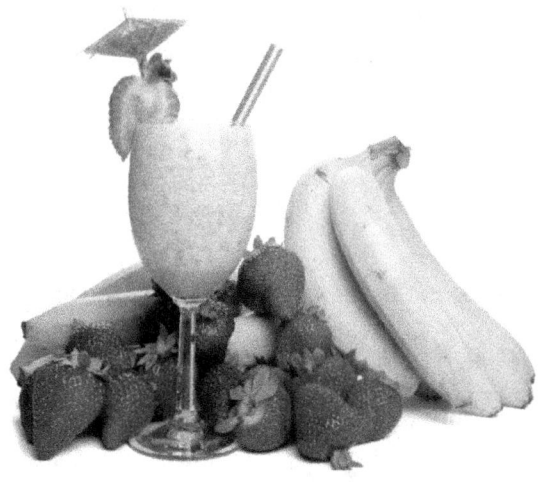

We are all well aware of the health benefits of fruit and vegetables. Yet, even with this information, many of us do not eat enough fruit and vegetables in our daily diets. One great way to increase our intake of fruits and vegetables is by drinking smoothies. They are delicious and packed full of vitamins and minerals. The major downside is that they can be quite expensive to buy. The best way around this is to make your own. There are hundreds of quick and easy recipes available on the internet, many of which use everyday fruit and vegetables which you will most likely already have at home.

So what makes the best blender for making smoothies? First of all, as mentioned in the previous chapter, it needs to be easy to clean. If a blender is not easy to clean, it is much less useful as it will not be convenient enough to use in everyday life. If you buy a blender which takes a long while to clean then chances are it will spend most of its life at the back of a cupboard gathering dust.

Secondly the bender must have enough power to do its job well without any problems. We also look for stylish design, good build quality, after sales support and overall reliability. So what would I recommend as the best blender for making smoothies? There are several excellent candidates for this title in a range of price brackets.

Braun Powermax Blender

One of the contenders is the Braun Powermax. This blender is well made, very reliable and works very well. It is large enough for you to make enough smoothies to last a few days and is so powerful that it can cope with any fruit or vegetable you can throw at it. It is also very versatile for other applications. It will chop ice with ease and is great for mixing soups. Braun is a well-respected manufacturer that always scores highly in terms of build quality and reliability. The Powermax is no exception.

The materials are robust and of high quality and they have been put together very well. Their customer service is excellent too. The styling is elegant if conventional. There are several adaptations which make this blender excellent for smoothies. The best of which is the specially designed lid which has holes that allow the addition of liquid whilst blending. Most smoothie recipes require the addition of a fruit juice to thin the consistency of the smoothie. With many juicers this means stopping the blender and removing the lid. The Powermax allows you to mix in the juice whilst the blender is running to create an excellent smoothie very quickly. It is also very easy to clean. The Powermax always scores highly in blender reviews.

Bosch Porsche Designer Blender

The next candidate is the Bosch Porsche Designer Blender. One of the main strengths of this blender is its stylish look. It will certainly not spend time at the back of a cupboard. Anyone familiar with Porsche Design products will know that they are always excellent. They are well built, perform well and look amazing, just like Porsche cars. This blender is no exception. It is definitely not just a pretty face. By teaming up with electrical giants Bosch, Porsche has created a product which looks great and also performs extremely well. This is a great all round blender and one of the very best available on the market with the added advantage of the wow factor. It looks great in any kitchen.

Breville Ikon Blender

Another of our favorite blenders is the Breville Ikon blender. This well designed and well-made blender is a great all-rounder. Not only is it great for smoothies, its vast array of speeds and settings make it suitable for a range of applications. The stainless steel which it is constructed from is of very high quality. The build quality is excellent and reliability is second to none. The revolutionary design of the blade allows the Ikon to closely hug the bowl and illuminate food traps. The design ensures a good quality, smooth final product with no lumps of unmixed fruit and ensures that the blender is easy to clean after use. The motor is very powerful and crushes ice with absolute ease.

There are many great blenders for making smoothies on the market and these are three of the very best. It is an excellent idea to buy a blender for making smoothies as it can make a real difference to the health and well-being of both yourself and your family, whilst also allowing you to save money and use up fruit and vegetables which otherwise would go to waste.

If you have children it can be very difficult to introduce enough healthy food into their diet. Many children will avoid fruit and vegetables and miss out on vital vitamins and minerals which their bodies need. As mentioned in Chapter 10, smoothies are a great way to persuade them to try these vital foods and vastly improve their diet. If you involve your child in the making of the smoothie he/she is very likely to drink the finished product. You will also be able to tailor the recipes to his/her specific tastes and you are in full control of exactly what goes into the drinks, unlike the products you buy from the supermarket.

A well designed blender can make it very simple to make your own smoothies at home, even if you have a busy lifestyle. If you do your research and purchase the best blender for making smoothies, you and your family will be drinking delicious, healthy homemade smoothies with maximum convenience.

ABOUT THE AUTHOR

Patricia Young is an individual that not only cares for her environment but also cares about what she puts into her body. She works in the field of sustainable development and is a strong supporter of organic products. As she was a "juicer" incorporating green smoothies into her diet was not a problem for her.

Her book on green smoothies outlines all the benefits of having a green smoothie and this includes using it to cleanse the body. There are also some great green smoothie recipes that the reader can try out to see how effective the process can be.